An Easy Way To Understand Your Body Systems

Also By Brian B Jacques

His very popular Series of Mini-Health Books includes:

- An Easy Way To Understand Eczema and Psoriasis
- An Easy Way To Understand Stress and Depression
- An Easy Way To Understand Vitamins and Minerals
- An Easy Way To Understand Parasites, Worms, Candida, Constipation & Detoxing
- An Easy Way To Understand Crohn's Disease and IBD
- An Easy Way To Understand Body Building For Men And Women
- An Easy Way To Understand Alzheimer's Disease
- An Easy Way To Understand Herpes
- An Easy Way To Understand Parkinson's Disease
- An Easy Way To Understand Autism
- An Easy Way To Understand Fibromyalgia
- An Easy Way To Understand Your Body Systems
- An Easy Way To Understand Erectile Dysfunction
- An Easy Way To Understand Heart Disease, High Blood Pressure & Stroke
- An Easy Way To Understand Detoxing For Men & Women
- How To Lose Weight After 40
- How To Lose Weight And Maintain Your Ideal Weight Permanently
- Amino Acids & Enzymes—What Are They & Why Do You Need Them
- The Little A–Z Dictionary of Herbal Remedies
- The Magic Of Vitamins & Minerals
- Effective Methods To Stop Smoking

All these books are available as Kindle Editions (available from the Kindle Store on Amazon.com, and other countries Amazon sites where the Kindle platform is supported.) Many of these books are also available for the Barnes and Noble "Nook". In addition, all these titles will shortly be available as print editions from the Amazon website. A downloadable eBook version will also available from the publishers website at www.wisdomforlifemedia.com

An Easy Way To Understand Your Body Systems

To Know Better – To Get Better With Natural Remedies

Brian B Jacques

Wisdom For Life Media

Publisher: Wisdom For Life Media (www.wisdomforlifemedia.com)

While they have made every effort to verify the information provided
in this publication, neither the author nor the publisher assumes any
responsibility for errors in, omissions from, or different interpretation of
the subject matter.

The information herein may be subject to varying laws, regulations, and
practices in different areas, states and countries. The purchaser or reader
assumes all responsibility for use of the information.

All information included within this book is for educational purposes
only. The author and publishers do not attempt to diagnose or treat any
medical conditions, be it to do with health, diet or exercise.

If you consider that you have any kind of medical condition, then, you
should consult a qualified medical practitioner or doctor before starting
any vitamin and/or mineral program or supplement regime, exercise or
health training program or diet suggested in this book.

This book is not intended for anyone under the age of 18 years, nor is it
intended for breast feeding or pregnant women, underweight people or
anyone with eating disorders or a health condition that requires special
diets or medical treatment.

The author and publishers disclaim any liability for any loss however
caused by anyone using the information contained in this book.

Images
All images are either copyright the author, or are used under the terms of
a Royalty Free License.

ISBN - 13: 978-1502313980
ISBN - 10: 1502313987

Published in The United States of America

"Education is the kindling of a flame, not the filling of a vessel." — Socrates

Contents

Acknowledgment

To my wife, Tatyana, whose constant love, presence and belief in me makes everything possible and worthwhile.

Introduction

In this latest book in my Mini Health Series, I want to discuss the body systems. I have put them into nine categories as follows:

- Circulatory
- Digestive
- Glandular
- Immune
- Intestinal
- Nervous
- Respiratory
- Structural
- Urinary

As you will see as you read through these systems, I have explained what important function each system performs in the body, as well as some lifestyle suggestions, and finally I have included some of the ailments that befall each system and some suggested natural herbal remedies and/or dietary supplements that have proved beneficial over the years.

No medications have been included in this book for the simple reason that I wanted to focus on alternative treatments. Here is one thing I always find interesting watching drug commercials on TV. There is almost more air-time spent on describing the side effects of the medication than what there is on describing the benefits. To me, that says a lot!

And finally, it is important to understand that each of the body systems is interrelated, therefore if there is a weakness in any one of the body systems, it will cause a malfunction in all the other body systems as well.

So let us make a start!

The Body Systems

The Circulatory System

Functions of the Circulatory System

Basic Function

The circulatory system is responsible for transporting nutrients to the cells and removing waste from the cells.

After the lungs have replaced the "blue" venal blood with red (by replacing carbon dioxide with oxygen), the heart pushes it throughout the body via arteries.

Arteries

Are living tubes with an outer layer of muscle. They allow for nutrient delivery to be adjusted according to the part of the body that needs it most. This causes a change in blood pressure in that area. Extreme nervous tension may cause a general vessel contraction that makes blood pressure soar, causing the heart to work harder.

Capillaries

Are the tiniest blood vessels. They carry blood to the areas of the body farthest from the heart.

Veins

Carry blood, now devoid of oxygen and full of carbon dioxide and other cell wastes, away for cleansing in the kidneys and re-oxygenation in the lungs. One complete cycle takes about 20 seconds. One-way valves in the leg veins help ease the heart's work.

The Lymphatic System

Is completely separate from the blood system. It is still part of the circulatory system because it re-circulates blood plasma trapped in tissue spaces. Lymph fluid not only helps to clear the tissue spaces but forms an important part of the immune system.

Common Problems Associated With The Circulatory System:

- Cholesterol/triglyceride buildup
- Hypertension
- Arterial plaque
- Stress
- Poor circulation
- Heart disease

Lifestyle Suggestions:

- Eat low to moderate amounts of fat daily.
- Avoid saturated fats.
- Eat lots of fruits, vegetables, onions and garlic.
- Perform aerobic exercise, especially walking.
- Manage weight.
- Avoid stress.

Interesting Facts:

- Cholesterol is made by the cells of all animals; humans manufacture most of their own in the liver. Cholesterol levels become dangerous when vessels are unprotected from oxidation by low levels of vitamin E and other antioxidants.

- A recent survey found that only 4 percent of women believe heart disease to be a top health risk, when in fact 34 percent die from this cause alone.

- According to the American Heart Association, 50 percent of middle-aged Americans have dangerously high levels of blood cholesterol.

Supplements for Circulatory System Health

For Cholesterol:
Chinese Red Yeast Rice

Chinese Red Yeast Rice has been used very effectively to lower cholesterol levels. This is due to it containing a family of monacolins (polyketides) with the ability to inhibit cholesterol synthesis and lower plasma cholesterol levels.

Garlic

Garlic is excellent for purging candida yeast and parasites from the body. Garlic has so many uses from using it in cooking to it being an excellent product for heart health. It also has antibacterial, anti-fungus and antiviral properties. Other recognized health benefits of garlic include, acting as an antibiotic and having anti-cholesterol and anti-hypertensive properties.

It is also an antioxidant which protects the body against the effects of free radical damage. Its high sulphur content assists in cell purification.

Allicin is the principle biological active compound which gives garlic its odor. Be warned. Many so called "odorless" garlic products have the active compound removed which makes it rather worthless. It can be obtained as a garlic bulb, in a capsule or in tablet form.

Lecithin

Lecithin is an important phospholipid which is needed and utilized by all body cells as well as the heart, liver and kidneys. As it is a fat itself, it adheres to cell and nerve linings, forming a slippery barrier to prevent cholesterol and other fats from sticking. This ensures that blood flows more freely.

For The Heart:
Co-QIO

Co-Q10 is essential for generating energy in every body cell and may help prevent heart disease and hypertension. Co-Q10 is also an antioxidant and is used in dental practices to help fight gum disease. Statins—cholesterol lowering drugs, destroy Co-Q10, so anyone taking these drugs should consider supplementing with Co-Q10.

Ginkgo Biloba

Ginkgo Biloba promotes increased circulation. It also dilates blood vessels and bronchioles to improve circulation and oxygenation of cells. It also has scientifically proven nervous-system benefits in addition to improving memory function.

Hawthorn Berries

Hawthorn Berries are known as the heart herb. It improves circulation and heart strength. In studies, hawthorn recipients also reported fewer overall symptoms, less fatigue and less shortness of breath.

Hawthorn Berries are often taken along with ginkgo biloba to improve circulation especially to the heart.

Magnesium

This essential mineral keeps the heart muscle from going into spasm.

For Vascular Problems:
(Varicose Veins, Hemorrhoids, Spider Veins)

Proanthocyanidins

Often sold under the trade name Pycnogenol. Proanthocyanidins are powerful antioxidants obtained from grape seed and pine bark. They help prevent cell damage by quenching oxidative free radicals. This combination of antioxidant nutrients has been shown to be many times more powerful than vitamin C or E. Proanthocyanidins also improve the integrity of collagen fibers, strengthening tissues in the skin, blood vessels, muscles, cartilage and other connective tissues.

Problems with Circulation:
(High Blood Pressure, Cold Hands and Feet, Hardening of the Arteries)

Capsicum

Capsicum also called cayenne has a warming effect and is often used to treat instances of cold hands and cold feet. As such it is an excellent circulatory product. It has also gained a good reputation as a painkiller and digestive aid. The main active ingredient is capsaicin—an oily phytochemical. Additionally, it has been used to relieve symptoms of a cold and sore throat.

Garlic

Garlic is excellent for purging candida yeast and parasites from the body. Garlic has so many uses from using it in cooking to it being an excellent product for heart health. It also has antibacterial, anti-fungus and antiviral properties. Other recognized health benefits of garlic include, acting as an antibiotic and having anti-cholesterol and anti-hypertensive properties.

It is also an antioxidant which protects the body against the effects of free radical damage. Its high sulphur content assists in cell purification.

Allicin is the principle biological active compound which gives garlic its odor. Be warned. Many so called "odorless" garlic products have the active compound removed which makes it rather worthless. It can be obtained as a garlic bulb, in a capsule or in tablet form.

Parsley

Parsley is probably one of the best known herbs as it is used in culinary dishes as well as for medicinal uses. It comes in a variety of different "leaf types", from feather like to curled to flat. The flat leafed variety is most often used for medicinal purposes.

It is used to treat urinary tract infections, indigestion, to relieve the effects of gas and as a digestive aid. Additionally, it is a natural body deodorizer and eradicates bad breath.

The Digestive System

Functions of the Digestive System

Basic Function

The basic function of the digestive system is the breakdown and assimilation of foods, primarily carbohydrates, fats and proteins:

- Protein into Amino Acids
- Carbohydrates into Sugar & Starches
- Fats into Fatty Acids

Stomach

Secretes some enzymes and hydrochloric acid (HCl) to break down protein. Within 2-6 hours, all food is emptied into the small intestine.

Small Intestine

Over 90 percent of digestion and absorption takes place here. The acid in the stomach is neutralized and food is mixed with enzymes, bile and pancreatic juices.

Liver

Aids in digestion and detoxification of food impurities and inspects nutrients before allowing them into the bloodstream.

Gallbladder

Stores bile used to break down dietary fat.

Pancreas

Produces digestive juices and helps control blood sugar.

Common Problems Associated With The Digestive System:

- Indigestion
- Heartburn
- Insufficient enzymes
- Stomach ulcers
- Stomach cramps

Lifestyle Suggestions:

- Avoid caffeine, alcohol and soft "sugary" drinks
- Eat raw fruits and vegetables rich in enzymes
- Avoid overeating

- Eat no later than 2-3 hours before bedtime
- Avoid resting after meals

Interesting Facts:

- 70-year-old's may produce as little as half the enzymes they produced when they were 20. By age 50, many people will produce only 15 percent of the hydrochloric acid (HCl) they did at age 25, and about a third of all people over the age of 65 secrete almost none

- Digestive problems cost the nation billions each year in medical bills and absence from work.

Supplements for Digestive System Health

For Acid and indigestion:

Papaya

Papaya contains proteolytic enzymes that aid in the digestion of proteins.

Peppermint

Peppermint stimulates the production of digestive fluids. It also eradicates bad breath and helps settle an upset stomach. If purchased in liquid form, then only tiny drops should be applied to water, otherwise it will be too strong.

Activated Charcoal

Absorbs poisons in the digestive tract. Activated Charcoal is one of the best remedies for arresting acute diarrhea, bloating, chemical poisoning, high cholesterol, foul belching and severe gas.

To Support the Liver:

Milk Thistle

This natural support to the liver contains a mixture of bioflavonoids, including silymarin. Milk Thistle strengthens the liver against autointoxication and stimulates protein synthesis in liver cells, which generates DNA and RNA.

For Under Acid Conditions, Heavy Feeling in the Stomach:

Korean Ginseng

Korean Ginseng—also called Panax Ginseng—has been used for over 5,000 years as a preventative tonic to nourish the whole body, especially for stress, fatigue and weak conditions. It grows primarily in China, South Korea and Japan.

Korean Ginseng is considered the strongest form of ginseng. Ginsenoside compounds assist in lowering blood sugar levels, while polysaccharides help to enhance the immune system. Korean Ginseng's antioxidant properties help to stimulate the immune system to help protect the body from various diseases and stress.

Korean Ginseng assists in the production of endorphins which makes a person feel exhilarated. It also has significant sexual health benefits to help improve erectile function, increase testosterone and sperm count.

Enzymes

If you are enzyme deficient (which most people are) due to a lack of enzymes in the food, or the way it is cooked and/or processed, then you can purchase a multi-enzyme product. Make sure though that there are no artificial fillers or additives in it. Enzymes are very important as they make things happen in the body. Without them, your body would not function at all.

The Glandular System

Functions of the Glandular System

Basic Function

Among their many functions, glands regulate emotions, promote growth, determine sexual identity, control body temperature and assist in the repair of damaged tissue.

Pituitary Gland

About the size of a pea, this gland resides in the brain and is often called the master gland because it secretes hormones that regulate virtually every other gland in the body.

Pineal Gland

The tiny pineal gland (also known as the third eye) is shaped like a pine cone and is located in the center of the brain. It secretes melatonin—a hormone that affects waking and sleep patterns. The production of melatonin is stimulated by darkness and inhibited by light.

When seen under X-rays the pineal gland is often calcified due in part to fluoride in drinking water and toothpaste.

The pineal gland is activated by daylight and controls various body functions in harmony with the hypothalamus gland.

The Hypothalamus Gland

One of the most important functions of the hypothalamus gland is to link the nervous system to the endocrine system via the pituitary gland (the master gland).

The hypothalamus gland secretes and synthesizes nerve hormones which in turn secrete or inhibit the secretion of pituitary hormones.

Body temperature is controlled by the hypothalamus gland, and it is also in charge of directing the body's emotions and feelings, such as: thirst, hunger, sexual desire as well as the biological clock that is responsible for determining the aging process.

Adrenal Glands

Situated atop the kidneys, these glands secrete several hormones. Adrenaline (epinephrine) is well-known: it stimulates the heart, keeps blood pressure normal and raises blood sugar levels. Along with making sex hormones, these glands secrete hormones that help regulate metabolism.

Thyroid Gland

This gland heavily influences growth and the metabolic rate (i.e., the level of activity within the body). That's why the thyroid should be checked when a person is either overweight or underweight. Located at the base of the front of the neck, it influences our motions, intellectual ability and physical vitality, and it was once considered our master gland.

Parathyroid Glands

Acting in concert with the thyroid in controlling the balance of calcium, these four pea-sized structures are attached to the back of the thyroid.

Thymus Gland

Butterfly-shaped and similar to the thyroid, the thymus is high in the chest behind the sternum (breast bone). Formed mostly of lymphatic tissue, it plays a key role in producing the immune system's T-cells (T stands for thymus). T-cells circulate in the blood and lymph to help protect the body from invaders or malignant cells.

Pancreas

This flat, yellow gland is about 5 inches long, residing just below the left side of the rib cage. It has two main functions: 1) to manufacture enzymes that help digest food, and 2) to secrete insulin, a hormone that helps regulate the amount of glucose (a type of sugar) in the blood. Glucose is used for energy.

Ovaries

Located on each side of the lower abdomen of women, these glands regulate the reproductive process through hormone secretions. Ovulation is the release of an egg from an ovary.

Testes

Located outside the body for better temperature control, they manufacture and store spermatozoa. They also produce testosterone, which controls the physical and mental characteristics of a male.

Common Problems Associated With The Glandular System:

- Hormone imbalance
- Emotional stress
- Reproductive troubles
- Hyper/hypo sugar levels

Lifestyle Suggestions:

- Eat regular, wholesome meals.
- Avoid smoking, alcohol and stimulants.
- Exercise regularly.
- Manage your stress.

Interesting Facts

- Every hormone is conveyed through either blood or lymph to stimulate or inhibit the activity of another organ or tissue.

- Prolonged stress can shrivel the thymus and lymph glands and exhaust the adrenals, which tire of trying to keep up with demand.

Supplements for Glandular System Health

Low Blood Sugar:
Licorice Root

Licorice has long been recognized for the natural sweetness of its deep-sinking roots. Next to ginseng, licorice is the most popular herb used in Chinese formulas. It helps support the adrenal glands during periods of stress.

High Blood Sugar – Diabetes:
Nopal

Nopal or Mexican Cactus as it is sometimes called is traditionally used by the Mexicans as a food especially in salads. The nutritional factors in nopal act in the bowel to prevent fat and excessive sugars from entering the bloodstream. By helping the body maintain balanced blood sugar levels, Nopal aids the body in its battle against obesity. Additionally, it is used as an anti-inflammatory, as a laxative and as a hypoglycemic vehicle for diabetes and gastritis.

Gymnema Sylvestre

Gymnema Sylvestre is a climbing plant which is native to Australia, part of Africa and central and southern India, and is used in Ayurvedic medicine. It is primarily used for weight management to control appetite and cravings, but has also been used to treat constipation and diabetes.

Chromium

Chromium is a trace mineral essential for proper pancreatic function. It assists in regulating insulin in the body and therefore has an effect on how much energy you get from your food. It helps to reduce food cravings and improves lifespan. It is also important for proper heart function.

Adrenal Exhaustion:
B Complex

B-vitamins are particularly important for the nervous system and are also vital for good digestive function and enzyme reactions that control energy, circulation, hormones and overall health. Since the same amount of each B vitamin is not necessarily needed by the body; this formula is usually balanced to assist B12 absorption.

Hypothyroidism:

Spirulina

Spirulina is a type of fresh-water blue-green algae composed of approximately 65-71 percent protein making it one of the richest vegetable sources of protein known. These proteins are biologically complete, containing all 8 essential amino acids in their proper ratios.

Much of the protein in spirulina is in the form of biliprotein which has been pre-digested by algae, making it 5 times easier to break down than either meat or soy protein. In fact, the digestibility of spirulina protein is rated 85 percent, compared to approximately 20 percent for beef protein.

This easy to digest type of protein is especially beneficial for those suffering from problems associated with excessive animal protein and refined foods intake—namely those with arthritis, cancer, diabetes, hypoglycemia, obesity, or similar degenerative conditions.

Kelp

Kelp is a brown algae that comes from the sea. It responds to sunlight and takes in minerals and other nutrients from the water. It is an excellent source of iodine. Iodine is needed for proper functioning of the thyroid and pituitary glands.

The thyroid is responsible for maintaining metabolism and body temperature. In fact during stressful periods, the thyroid can work overtime to try and normalize body functions, therefore supplementing with kelp can be very beneficial for boosting energy.

A proper functioning metabolism is also important for maintaining weight control, which can sometimes be a problem when the body is under stress, and a person is susceptible to "binge eat" on comfort foods.

Supplements for Glandular System Health - Female

Menstrual:
Dong Quai

Dong Quai—a member of the celery family—is one of the oldest known herbs, having been used in China, Japan and Korea for over 1,000 years. It is primarily known as a women's product, to relieve menopausal symptoms such as: hot flashes, menstrual disorders such as cramps, irregular menstrual cycles, infrequent periods, premenstrual syndrome (PMS), and menopausal symptoms.

It is suggested that Dong Quai contains compounds that may help reduce pain, dilate blood vessels, and stimulate and relax uterine muscles.

In traditional Chinese medicine (TCM), different parts of the dong quai root are used for different actions in the body: the root head is used as an anticoagulant, the main part of the root is used as a tonic, and the tail-end of the root is used to remove blood stagnation. Because it is a balancer of the female hormonal system, it is often called "females ginseng."

Menopause:
Black Cohosh

Black Cohosh is widely used to treat menopausal symptoms such as hot flashes, night sweats, migraines, mood swings, heart palpitations and dryness. The roots of the plant are used medically and are available as capsules, a liquid extract or tablets.

Pregnancy:
Red Raspberry

This herb is renowned for its nutritional support of the female reproductive system. Red Raspberry is known to nourish and strengthen the uterus. A common backyard fruit bush, Red Raspberry is an excellent herbal source of iron, manganese and niacin. It also contains quantities of vitamins C, A, D, E and B, as well as phosphorus and calcium.

Desire: Infertility:
Maca

Maca, also known as Peruvian Ginseng is used to increase stamina, energy and sexual function in both men and women. In one study, researchers found that maca may help alleviate sexual dysfunction caused by the use of selective-serotonin re-uptake inhibitors (SSRIs) which are used in the treatment of depression.

Supplements for Glandular System Health - Male

Benign Prostatic Hyperplasia (BPH)
Saw Palmetto

Saw palmetto is mainly used to treat benign prostatic hyperplasia (BPH). BPH is a male condition which includes frequent urination, difficulty in fulfilling the urge to urinate, dribbling after urination, a weak urinary stream, and finally, waking up several times at night to urinate.

Erectile Dysfunction
Yohimbe

A native to the Congo, Cameroon, Nigeria, and Gabon, yohimbe is used to prevent depression as it inhibits monoamine oxidase (MAO). Additionally it is used to treat erectile dysfunction either as a single herb, or in combination with other herbs.

Korean Ginseng

Korean Ginseng—also called Panax Ginseng - has been used for over 5,000 years as a preventative tonic to nourish the whole body, especially for stress, fatigue and weak conditions. It grows primarily in China, South Korea and Japan.

Korean Ginseng is considered the strongest form of ginseng. Ginsenoside compounds assist in lowering blood sugar levels, while polysaccharides help to enhance the immune system. Korean Ginseng's antioxidant properties help to stimulate the immune system to help protect the body from various diseases and stress.

Korean Ginseng assists in the production of endorphins which makes a person feel exhilarated. It also has significant sexual health benefits to help improve erectile function, increase testosterone as well as sperm count.

Maca

Maca, also known as Peruvian Ginseng is used to increase stamina, energy and sexual function in both men and women.

The Immune System

Functions of the Immune System

Basic Function

The Immune System provides specialized fighting forces that are tailor-made to combat internal invasions, whether they are microbes or toxic chemicals. It also provides "security patrols" that police the body; these are stationed in lymph nodes, openings of the body and other strategic locations.

Inside the body, a trillion highly specialized cells will launch an unending battle against alien organisms. Within minutes the immune system will sense an enemy's presence and send out scavenger cells, which immediately attack the invaders.

Remember that during any war, there are great "expenses" involved. That translates into a greater than normal requirement for better nutrition, and rest to conserve energy.

Bone Marrow

Produces B cells that produce antibodies—foot soldiers of the system. Antibodies neutralize foreign invaders.

Lymph

Is blood serum that has leaked from the bloodstream into the tissue spaces and is recovered by a network of tiny vessels that separate it from the bloodstream. This fluid brings with it tissue, toxins and microbes.

Lymph Nodes

Are gathering points throughout the body where lymph travels to unload toxins and microbes for cleansing.

Tonsils

Are lymph tissue in the throat guarding the respiratory and digestive systems.

Thymus

Located behind the breast bone. This central gland of the lymphatic system helps "train" part of the army of B-cells to convert them into T-cells. T-cells are highly specialized cells which play a crucial role in destroying foreign invaders—especially tumor cells in the body.

Spleen

A lymphatic gland under the left ribs, the spleen helps filter the blood and is a pumping aid for lymph fluids throughout the body. It is involved in the production of white blood cells.

Common Problems Associated With The Immune System:

- Viral/bacterial attack
- Fatigue
- Stress
- Cancer
- AIDS

Lifestyle Suggestions:

- Reduce stress.
- Eat lots of fruits and vegetables.
- Eat adequate complete proteins.
- Avoid simple sugars.
- Get adequate sleep and exercise.

Interesting Facts:

- Immunity comes from the word "immunis," a Latin word meaning "safe." In any given year, roughly 50 percent of Americans will catch a cold, and 40 percent will get the flu. 80 percent of all illnesses can be traced to stress.

- Your whole personal immune army weighs about two pounds and consists of about a trillion cells assisted by 100 quintillion antibody molecules.

Supplements for Immune System Health

Bacteria, Virus, Fungus:

Garlic

This popular herb offers a boost to the immune system with its antibacterial, antifungal and antiviral properties.

Garlic has many uses:
- Anti-biotic - natural penicillin
- Arteriosclerosis
- Arthritis
- Asthma
- Blood poisoning
- High blood pressure
- Anti-viral
- Anti-bacterial
- Destroys many types of parasites
- For respiratory conditions use with mullein or lobelia
- As a decongestant / expectorant use with lobelia
- For bacterial infection use with golden seal, echinacea, Pau d'Arco
- For viral infection use with colloidal silver
- For yeast infections use with Pau d'Arco
- For swollen lymph nodes use with lobelia and mullein
- For parasites use with pumpkin seeds and black walnut

Colloidal Silver

Colloidal silver has many uses and has been found to be effective against many surface and internal micro-organisms, viruses, protozoa, amoeba, fungi, parasites and yeasts. It works by in-activating the enzyme that is responsible for the multiplication of many of these invaders.

There are many different colloidal silver products on the market. You need to source one that contains 99.9 percent pure silver, without any additives, apart from purified water.

Echinacea

Echinacea contains polysaccharides that stimulate the production of phagocytes (cells that engulf and consume foreign matter) and activate T-lymphocytes, macrophages and natural killer cells. Taken at the earliest sign of a cold or infection, echinacea may help cut recovery time considerably.

Olive Leaf Extract

Olive Leaf Extract supports normal blood pressure and cholesterol levels and strengthens the immune system against viral and bacterial attacks.

Una de Gato (Cats Claw)

- The bark of a vine from South America. Una de Gato provides beneficial alkaloids to stimulate the immune system. It is also used for the following:
- As a cancer therapy to reduce the side effects of chemotherapy.
- As an anti-inflammatory for all types of arthritis
- As a bowel and stomach protector and cleanser, and to treat ulcerative colitis as well as stomach ulcers.
- To treat a variety of bowel problems including, but not limited to: Crohn's disease, diverticulitis and irritable bowel syndrome (IBS).
- An excellent general body tonic to tone and protect all body systems.
- It is usually taken in capsule form.

Elderberry

One of the oldest known herbs. It works in the respiratory and immune body systems, and is usually used to counter the effects of colds, flu, congestion, sore throat and inflammation.

Zinc Lozenges

Zinc is often combined with Echinacea and Licorice Root (as a natural sweetener) to treat the effects of a sore throat or other mouth infections. It also supplies excellent immune system support.

When buying this type of product, make sure there are no artificial fillers or artificial sugar coatings which would be used as a sweetener.

Pau D'Arco

Pau D'Arco is native to South America. It contains a chemical called lapachol, which may provide nutritional support to the immune system. It is commonly used against many conditions of unwanted growth, including fungus, yeast and tumors as well as fungal infections. Historically, it has also been used to remedy the side effects of some antibiotics.

It is available as a capsule, tablet or as a lotion.

Bifidophilus

A probiotic supplement. Bifidophilus products contain living organisms from various strains of "friendly" bacteria to help replace depleted bacteria in the colon. They are necessary for proper immune function, and to help balance the digestive system.

Probiotics are very beneficial after taking a course of antibiotics. Antibiotics not only kill foreign invaders, but they kill "friendly" bacteria too.

Vitamin C

The common cold and flu are viral infections. If you increase your intake of vitamin C by taking a high dose supplement then your cold will clear up much quicker. Vitamin C is also water soluble so it is easily depleted in the body.

Compromised Immune System:
Una de Gato (Cats Claw)

- The bark of a vine from South America. Una de Gato provides beneficial alkaloids to stimulate the immune system. It is also used for the following:
- As a cancer therapy to reduce the side effects of chemotherapy.
- As an anti-inflammatory for all types of arthritis.
- As a bowel and stomach protector and cleanser, and to treat ulcerative colitis as well as stomach ulcers.
- To treat a variety of bowel problems including, but not limited to: Crohn's disease, diverticulitis and irritable bowel syndrome (IBS).
- An excellent general body tonic to tone and protect all body systems.
- It is usually taken in capsule form.

Free Radical Damage:
Proanthocyanidins

Often sold under the trade name Pycnogenol. Proanthocyanidins are powerful antioxidants obtained from grape seed and pine bark. They help prevent cell damage by quenching oxidative free radicals. This combination of antioxidant nutrients has been shown to be many times more powerful than vitamin C or E. Proanthocyanidins also improve the integrity of collagen fibers, strengthening tissues in the skin, blood vessels, muscles, cartilage and other connective tissues.

Any Other Antioxidants

There are antioxidant vitamins: vitamins A, C and E, and Beta Carotene, antioxidant minerals: selenium and zinc, and antioxidant herbs: garlic, ginkgo biloba and many others have antioxidant properties. All provide protection against free radical damage. Unless there are other health issues where specific herbal products may be required, which would provide some antioxidant protection, the usual way to help protect the body against the effects of free radical damage is to take an antioxidant vitamin and mineral supplement.

The Intestinal System

Functions of the Intestinal System

Basic Function

The intestines comprise the small intestine, large intestine and the rectum. The small intestine is approximately 20 feet long and about one inch in diameter. Its function is to absorb the nutrients from food through velvety tissue called villi.

The large intestine (or colon) is approximately five feet long and approximately three inches in diameter. Water is absorbed from waste which then creates a stool. The stool enters the rectum where nerve impulses create the urge to eliminate it.

Small Intestine

Over 90 percent of digestion and absorption takes place here. The acid from the stomach is neutralized, and food is mixed with enzymes, bile and pancreatic juices. The small intestine is usually considered part of the digestive system, since almost all nutrients are processed and absorbed by the time a meal reaches the large intestine.

Large Intestine

Also called the colon or lower bowel. It is divided into three parts: ascending (from the end of the small intestine near the appendix, up the abdominal cavity on the right side); transverse (crossing just under the ribs in front of the stomach); and descending (down the left side to the rectum). Acting as a "compactor," the large intestine is aided by the presence and pressure of undigested fiber. This compacting action tends to cleanse the inner walls of the intestine, and during this squeezing, water is withdrawn, with a few ounces left to help prevent constipation.

The Ileocecal Valve

Is a muscle that opens to allow food to pass to the large intestine and then closes to prevent any from traveling back in the wrong direction. With different bacteria present in these areas, this valve keeps them in the right places.

The Appendix

Is lymph tissue that guards against infection. When it is weakened, it may become infected, swell or burst, endangering life.

The Rectum

The last five inches of the colon, ends with the anus, a powerful muscle which controls evacuation.

Common Problems Associated With The Intestinal System:

- Constipation/diarrhea
- Hemorrhoids
- Diverticulitis
- Colitis
- Crohn's disease
- Irritable bowel syndrome

Lifestyle Suggestions:

- Make sure you get adequate fiber in your diet
- Exercising can stimulate the intestinal system to work properly
- Avoid high fat foods
- Avoid foods containing excessive amounts of sugar
- Eat plenty of fresh fruits and vegetables

Interesting Fact:

- You may house 400 species and 100 trillion bacteria in your colon. Some of them synthesize vitamin K, B12 and biotin. Others (Friendly Flora) neutralize toxins and help control dangerous bacteria.

Supplements for Intestinal System Health

Diarrhea:
Bentonite (montmorillonite) Clay

Bentonite clay is very quick acting as it has the ability to bind the stools together. It does this by binding irritants in the gastrointestinal tract. One option is to combine the bentonite clay with a small quantity of apple sauce to make the clay more palatable. Apple sauce contains pectin—another binding agent. Incidentally pectin is also used in jam making to make the fruit "set".

Activated Charcoal

Charcoal is highly absorbent. Activated Charcoal can help in cases of poisoning or severe diarrhea as it absorbs irritants and toxins in the digestive tract. It may also help lower cholesterol levels as well as relieving the effects of foul belching and severe smelly gas. An alternative to activated charcoal is to use bentonite clay.

Constipation:
Psyllium

An excellent source of dietary fiber. Psyllium is gluten free and is therefore a useful fiber source for those suffering from celiac disease or gluten intolerance.

It expands dramatically from the size of the original seeds and it is therefore essential to drink plenty of water with this product.

Psyllium absorbs toxins from the intestinal tract and binds them to fecal matter for elimination.

As it is a bulking agent, it often gives a feeling of fullness and discourages a person from over eating.

One of the main causes of constipation is a lack of fiber in the diet.

Magnesium

This essential mineral can act as a laxative for a spastic colon (cramping and/or explosive bowel movement, sometimes caused by stress). Some over-the-counter laxatives contain magnesium. It is often combined with calcium to aid the structural system as well as helping relax the nervous system.

B Complex

Where spastic constipation is stress related, a B Complex vitamin supplement may be required along with vitamin C. B vitamins and vitamin C are water soluble and are easily depleted when the body is under stress. They are often referred to as the stress vitamins. Note. All the B vitamins work together so it is usually preferable to take a B Complex supplement and then top-up with individual B vitamins as required.

Parasites:

Black Walnut

Traditionally used as a nutritional aid for the intestinal system, Black Walnut has the same laxative action as cascara sagrada, but it works more gently. Due to its astringent qualities, Black Walnut has the power to assist the body in protecting itself from harmful agents such as parasitic worms. It also has a high iodine content, which is good for energy as it supports thyroid function.

Bifidophilus

A probiotic supplement. Bifidophilus products contain living organisms from various strains of "friendly" bacteria to help replace depleted bacteria in the colon. They are necessary for proper immune function, and to help balance the digestive system.

Probiotics are very beneficial after taking a course of antibiotics. Antibiotics not only kill foreign invaders, but they kill "friendly" bacteria too.

The Nervous System

Functions of the Nervous System

Basic Function

The basic function of the nervous system is to trigger and monitor all communication process in the body.

While the brain is the master controller, the nervous system also has local control points. For example, a burn reflex travels to and from the spinal cord so you withdraw your hand before your brain knows what happened.

There are three types of neurons: sensory neurons, which receive stimuli and carry impulses to the central nervous system (CNS); inter-neurons, which connect two or more neurons; and motor-neurons, which carry impulses away from the CNS to muscles or glands.

Impulses travel from one nerve cell to another across a space between them called a synapse with the help of chemical transmitters. Among these are acetylcholine, nor-epinephrine and serotonin.

Neuron

A nerve cell that includes receiving and transmitting arms that link it to billions of nerve cells throughout the body.

Neurotransmitter

One of several types of chemical messengers.

Brain

As master controller (and weighing an average of three pounds), it uses 20 percent of the body's total energy supply to power an estimated 10 billion brain cells.

Central Nervous System

The brain and spinal cord

Peripheral Nervous System

A network of nerves branching out from the spinal cord throughout the body.

Common Problems Associated With The Nervous System:

- Headaches
- Insomnia
- Nervous disorders
- Depression
- Memory dysfunction

Lifestyle Suggestions:

- Eat regular, wholesome meals.
- Avoid smoking, alcohol and stimulants.
- Exercise regularly.
- Manage your stress.
- Eat lots of green, leafy vegetables, fruits, whole grains and nuts.

Interesting Facts:

- Some nerve fibers can conduct nerve impulses as fast as 200 yards per second.

- Scientists are investigating evidence that dead nerve cells can be replaced by the body, a process once thought to be impossible.

- Prescriptions for antidepressants have increased over 100 percent in the last five years.

- To combat anxiety, a daily walk may be as effective as tranquilizers.

Supplements for Nervous System Health

Stress:
B Complex and Vitamin C

When the body is under stress, a B Complex vitamin supplement may be required along with vitamin C. B vitamins and vitamin C are water soluble and are easily depleted from the body, especially during stressful times. All the B vitamins work together so it is usually preferable to take a B Complex supplement and then top-up with individual B vitamins as required. The B vitamins and vitamin C are often referred to as the stress vitamins.

Depression:
St. John's Wort

This popular herb has gained national attention for its ability to alleviate mild to moderate depression. It contains an active constituent, hypericin, which appears to prolong the activity of serotonin (a neurotransmitter) in the brain. St. John's Wort may also lengthen the performance of dopamine and nor-epinephrine, two brain chemicals that are linked to depression. In Europe, many doctors prescribe this herb instead of prescription antidepressant drugs.

Note! You can find further details on Stress and Depression by reading my book "*An Easy Way to Understand Stress and Depression*", which is available from the Kindle Store at amazon. com, or the other Amazon country sites which support the Kindle Store. If you have a Barnes and Noble "Nook", then you can download this version from the Nook Press store. Also, there is a download printable version available at www.wisdomforlifemedia.com.

Mind, Memory Loss, Poor Memory:
Ginkgo Biloba

Ginkgo Biloba promotes increased circulation. It also dilates blood vessels and bronchioles to improve circulation and oxygenation of cells. It also has scientifically proven nervous-system benefits in addition to improving memory function.

The Respiratory System

Functions of the Respiratory System

Basic Function

The basic function of the respiratory system is to supply the body with oxygen and eliminate its by-product, carbon dioxide.

Fresh air is literally sucked into the body when the diaphragm muscle pulls down inside the chest cavity.

Traveling down the throat into the bronchial tubes, air branches out into the lungs and finally into 300 million tiny alveoli sacs. There, blood flowing close to the inner surface of the lungs exchanges fresh air with carbon dioxide and other waste gases, which are exhaled. Deep breathing makes it all happen more efficiently.

All along these air passages are millions of cilia, about 200 per cell, which help carry foreign particles and toxic mucus out of the lungs, throat and nasal cavities. Cilia move these particles in only one direction, unless they (the cilia) are poisoned by toxins like tobacco smoke. For those irritants that remain, immune cells are stationed in the area to engulf and dissolve these small intruders.

Mucus exuded by surface tissues of the respiratory and digestive tract keep respiratory tissues from dehydrating and cracking, in addition, they also have an antiseptic action.

When the body is too toxic, this waste spills over into other areas like the mucus of the respiratory system. This can cause irritation and swelling, and becomes a breeding ground for millions of unwelcome bacteria and viruses.

Sinuses

Here air is both warmed and moisturized for more efficient transfer of gases in the lungs.

Larynx

Air flows past the larynx (voice box) and into the bronchi on its way to the lungs.

Trachea

Also known as the windpipe, it leads to the bronchi.

Bronchi

The trachea leads into these, which subdivide into smaller and smaller passageways, the bronchioles.

Lungs

Within the lungs' air sacs, oxygen trades places with carbon dioxide or other gases that the body considers waste.

Diaphragm

This acts as the body's bellows to push and pull the air you breathe.

Common Problems Associated With The Respiratory System:

- Asthma
- Hay fever
- Cough
- Bronchitis

Lifestyle Suggestions:

- Do not smoke
- Avoid inhaling other people's smoke
- Make sure your digestive system is working properly
- Make sure your immune system is not compromised
- Eat plenty of fresh fruits and vegetables
- Get plenty of exercise
- Make sure you get adequate rest and sleep

Interesting Facts:

- The total respiratory surface is 25-50 times the surface area of your entire body.

- Non-smokers who are in close proximity to smokers raise their risk for lung cancer by 30 percent.

- Non-smokers in heavy vehicular traffic may breathe-in as many airborne free radical particles as a pack-a-day smoker.

Supplements for Respiratory System Health

Deficient Mucus (yellow & Thick), With a Dry Irritated Cough:

Mullein

Mullein has both mucilant and astringent properties. Its powerful healing abilities make it useful for healing weak lung tissue and chronic respiratory congestion. It has proven expectorant action that likely arises from saponin compounds in the plant. Scientific studies suggest that the mucilage in mullein protects mucous membranes, preventing cell invasion by viral allergens.

Excess Mucus (white, clear or watery mucus):

Fenugreek

Fenugreek is a respiratory system herb which assists in expelling mucous, phlegm and infections from the lungs, and toxic waste through the lymphatic system. In addition, fenugreek is able to dissolve a hardened build-up of mucous which can then be eliminated.

Garlic

A powerful, aromatic herb, garlic aids decongestion and expectoration. Garlic works especially well on lung congestion. It has known antibacterial and antiviral properties.

Echinacea

There are various strains of Echinacea. It is used to support the immune system and is involved in the production of white blood cells, which assists the body to fight infection. Echinacea purges toxins from the blood and enhances lymphatic drainage.

Golden Seal

Golden seal has infection-fighting abilities and anti-inflammatory properties, especially in the mucus membranes. It is sometimes combined with Echinacea and garlic to make a really powerful treatment for colds, flu and to treat other infections.

Asthma – caused by anxiety or stress:

Lobelia

Lobelia has a lengthy history of use as a herbal remedy for

respiratory conditions such as asthma, bronchitis, pneumonia, and cough. Traditionally, Native Americans smoked lobelia as a treatment for asthma. Today, some herbalists use lobelia to help clear mucus from the respiratory tract, including the throat, lungs, and bronchial tubes. Additionally, lobelia is used as part of a comprehensive treatment plan for asthma.

Asthma – due to a history of hay fever or respiratory allergies:

Alfalfa

Alfalfa is a grass which contains all the essential amino acids as well as being rich in trace minerals and enzymes. It is frequently taken to lessen the effects of hay fever allergies. It is also fed to horses as a counter to arthritic conditions and digestive problems.

As it is a good source of fiber, it is useful for detoxifying the body in addition to improving liver health.

Methyl Sulfonyl Methane (MSM)

Methyl Sulfonyl Methane is a sulfur dietary supplement that starts life in the sea. Plankton in the sea release sulfur compounds which rise into the atmosphere where ultra violet light converts them into MSM and DMSO (dimethyl sulfoxide)—a precursor to MSM.

MSM and DMSO return to earth attached to rain droplets. MSM is found in grains, vegetables, fruits, meat and poultry.

MSM is an organic form of sulfur that is found in living tissues. MSM is the only dietary supplement that relieves allergies and arthritic conditions at the same time. In the structural system it is an excellent treatment for arthritis, muscle pains, bursitis. Additionally it supports connective tissue such as ligaments, tendons, and muscle.

Sulfur is an important element in maintaining good health. But it is lacking in the Western diet. Therefore it would be worth considering as a preventative product.

Proanthocyanidins

Often sold under the trade name Pycnogenol. Proanthocyanidins are powerful antioxidants obtained from grape seed and pine bark. They help prevent cell damage by quenching oxidative free radicals.

This combination of antioxidant nutrients has been shown to be many times more powerful than vitamin C or E. Proanthocyanidins also improve the integrity of collagen fibers, strengthening tissues in the skin, blood vessels, muscles, cartilage and other connective tissues.

Alcohol Withdrawal:
Kudzu / St John's Wort

Historically Asian-healers have used Kudzu to treat colds, flu, high blood pressure, allergies and many other ailments.

More recently, Chinese-healers have used Kudzu to treat people who have an alcohol dependency. It has also been used with St John's Wort to treat the depressive effects of alcohol withdrawal. Kudzu is available in capsules, tablets, and as a dried root.

Stopping Smoking:
Lobelia / St John's Wort

Lobelia is used in a smoking prevention regime due to one of its active ingredients—lobeline which reduces the effects of nicotine in the body; especially the release of dopamine. Dopamine plays many important functions in the brain—especially with regard to drug addiction.

Lobelia is sometimes combined with St John's Wort to reduce the depressive and stress effects when a person is trying to give us smoking.

The two herbs provide a cleansing and detoxifying action, in addition to helping clear "tar" from the lungs—one of the health consequences of smoking.

The Structural System

Functions of the Structural System

Basic Function

The basic function of the skeleton is to provide support and protection for the body. The skeletal structure is so important that without it, you would end up in a heap on the floor.

The skeleton comprises all the bones in the body as well as some tissues including cartilage, ligaments and tendons that connect them.

In addition, the skeleton provides protection for internal organs: the heart, lungs, brain, eyes and spinal cord.

While teeth are considered part of the skeletal system, they are not made of bone. They are made of enamel and dentine. Enamel is by far the strongest substance in the human body.

Bones

Along with providing a strong foundation to support-or protect-other body parts, the body's 206 bones are living structures that manufacture new blood cells within the marrow. Minerals packed in protein sacs are "glued" together to make healthy bones stronger than iron. Physical activity stimulates the bones to maintain their strength. Bones provide a storehouse for minerals that can be withdrawn in emergencies.

Muscles

Attached to the bones are ligaments that hold bones together and tendons that connect bones to a total of 620 muscles. In addition to moving the body, they produce heat, squeeze blood into isolated tissues, maintain posture and, when exercised, increase endorphin hormones, which results in a feeling of well-being. Muscle tissue surrounds arteries so blood pressure can be increased where tissue nutrients are most needed.

Skin

The skin is the largest organ of the body-and the most exposed. It is a supple, elastic tissue that conserves heat and moisture. It is the first organ to respond to pain or touch. Skin also functions as a cooling system and helps regulate internal body temperature. Skin helps eliminate toxic matter through perspiration and reabsorbs its own surface oils irradiated by the sun in order to make vitamin D.

Hair

Hair follicles can be found almost everywhere in the skin. These are oiled from imbedded sebaceous glands, which keep the skin supple and waterproof. Hair is made of keratin protein and helps control body temperature. The root is the only living part and appears to draw toxic metals out of the blood, encapsulating them in dead hair cells that are pushed out of the skin. While hair also protects the body, a nerve attached to each follicle increases the body's sensitivity to touch.

Common Problems Associated With The Structural System:

- Arthritis
- Osteoporosis
- Muscle cramps
- Poor posture

Lifestyle Suggestions:

- Eat regular, balanced meals.
- Get adequate sources of calcium.
- Perform weight-bearing exercises, including walking.
- Chew fibrous fruits and vegetables for strong teeth.
- Practice good oral hygiene.

Interesting Facts:

- There are 100,000 strands of hair on the average head.

- Muscle tissue comprises about 40 percent of your body weight.

- Bedridden patients have been known to lose as much as one percent of their inner bone per week.

Supplements for Structural System Health

Joint Inflammation:

Alfalfa

Alfalfa is a grass which contains all the essential amino acids as well as being rich in trace minerals and enzymes. It is used to reduce joint inflammation in humans as well as in animals – especially horses.

Methyl Sulfonyl Methane (MSM)

Methyl Sulfonyl Methane is a sulfur dietary supplement that starts life in the sea. Plankton in the sea release sulfur compounds which rise into the atmosphere where ultra violet light converts them into MSM and DMSO (dimethyl sulfoxide)—a precursor to MSM.

MSM and DMSO return to earth attached to rain droplets. MSM is found in grains, vegetables, fruits, meat and poultry.

MSM is an organic form of sulfur that is found in living tissues. MSM is the only dietary supplement that relieves allergies and arthritic conditions at the same time. In the structural system it is an excellent treatment for arthritis, muscle pains, bursitis. Additionally it supports connective tissue such as ligaments, tendons, and muscle.

Sulfur is an important element in maintaining good health. But it is lacking in the Western diet. Therefore it would be worth considering as a preventative product.

Glucosamine

Glucosamine is a building block of cartilage. As such, it helps relieve symptoms of arthritis and restores cartilage health. By supplementing with glucosamine, it is possible to strengthen and rebuild cartilage throughout the body

Chondroitin

Chondroitin attracts fluid into the joints, where it acts as a shock absorber during impact. This fluid also brings vital nutrients to the cartilage. Chondroitin protects the cartilage from premature disintegration.

It is available in supplement form with glucosamine. Additionally, it can also be obtained as a glucosamine, chondroitin and MSM supplement.

Skin Problems:
Evening Primrose Oil

Evening Primrose Oil assists the body in producing prostaglandins. Evening Primrose Oil provides omega-6 essential fatty acids that help with such conditions as eczema and brittle nails.

Eczema & Psoriasis:
Pau D'Arco Lotion

Herbalists have long used Pau d'Arco to enhance and fortify the human immune system. Pau d'Arco Lotion is specially formulated for topical use on rashes on the hands, arms and face. The emollient properties of Pau d'Arco leave skin feeling smooth and supple.

Acne:
Tea Tree Oil

A native of Australia. Tea Tree Oil has many uses. It is highly prized for its antiseptic and anti-bacterial benefits. It is used to treat acne, athlete's foot, abscesses, boils, dandruff and Pyorrhea. It is also used to sterilize cuts,

Bone Health and Hair, Skin and Nails:
Horsetail

This herb has diuretic properties and can help with some kidney conditions. It is particularly effective for healing when blood is present in the urine. Horsetail also has astringent properties and as such, is used for bed-wetting in children and incontinence in Adults.

Horsetail is rich in silica, which helps to soothe and strengthen connective tissue. Silica is required for bone and cartilage formation, as well as assisting the body in absorbing and utilizing calcium. Calcium is needed for repairing fractures and treating bone diseases, including rickets and osteoporosis. Horsetail is used to strengthen bones, teeth, nails and hair. Improvements in cartilage formation helps to lessen inflammation and combat joint pain, arthritis, gout, muscle cramps, hemorrhoids, spasms and rheumatism.

The silica content in horsetail also promotes the growth of collagen—a protein found in connective tissue, Collagen assists in improving skin health and tone.

Calcium

Calcium is one of the most crucial minerals the body needs. As well as building strong teeth and bones, it is important in regulating muscle contractions which includes the heart beat. It also ensures that blood clots normally when you receive a cut. It is also an important mineral for maintaining the correct acid / alkaline balance

When taking calcium as a supplement, it is preferable to take it in a combination form of calcium and magnesium. Vitamin D should also be in the formula as it helps with the absorption of calcium. Also important is phosphorus, which works with calcium, boron, copper, and zinc (an antioxidant mineral).

Magnesium

Magnesium helps convert food to energy and makes sure that the parathyroid glands (which produce hormones to promote bone health) are working normally. It is also important for bones and teeth, as well as for the heart and nervous system. It is important for calcium uptake as well as being an anti-inflammatory mineral.

Vitamin D

Vitamin D helps regulate the amounts of calcium and phosphorous in the body. These substances help keep teeth and bones healthy.

Most of the vitamin D is made in the skin because of its reaction to sunlight. Incidentally, most people—and especially children—lack vitamin D either through a lack of sun exposure, or it is lacking in the diet.

In children, vitamin D is important for proper growth and development. It is also important for the synthesis of calcium. Anyone who is pregnant or breast-feeding should supplement with vitamin D. Older people especially should take a vitamin D supplement. Individuals who eat no meat or oily fish, rarely go outdoors or cover up when you do should also supplement with vitamin D.

The Urinary System

.

Functions of the Urinary System

Basic Function

After the body has adsorbed nutrients from the food, waste products are created which circulate in the blood and in the colon. The urinary system works in harmony with the lungs, skin, and intestines—all of which also excrete wastes—to keep the chemicals and water in the body balanced.

Urea is one type of waste the urinary system removes. Urea is created when certain proteins from meat and poultry and specific vegetables are broken down in the body. This waste material is then carried through the bloodstream to the kidneys for filtration.

More than 2 million filters in the kidneys separate toxic elements and excessive amounts of nutrients that cannot be stored or utilized (including water) from the blood.

The kidneys adjust the blood's pH by maintaining the proper sodium/ potassium balance necessary for each cell to make energy. These organs can even secrete hormones to help regulate the body.

After the kidneys extract just enough water to keep the body healthy, urine flows down a ureter (tube) into the bladder for storage. From there, it empties through another tube (urethra) to the outside.

Kidneys

Two kidneys reside behind the stomach, nestled in a protective cushion of fat. When they are inflamed, the kidneys ache and some people mistake this for a backache. But this backache can occur during any severe battle the body is waging in which lots of toxins are being processed which results in overloading the kidneys' ability to filter them out, thus actually tiring and poisoning the kidneys themselves.

Ureter

Attached to the bottom of each kidney, these tubes carry urine into the bladder.

Bladder

Urine is stored here. After it builds up, nerves signal the brain that it's time to be emptied. Holding urine too long in the bladder can encourage bacterial growth or cause chemical irritation.

Common Problems Associated With The Urinary System:

- Bladder/kidney infection
- Kidney stones
- Incontinence
- Cystitis
- Pain and irritation

Lifestyle Suggestions:

- Drink 64 oz. of water daily.
- Drink unsweetened cranberry juice.
- Eat lots of fruits and vegetables.
- Practice good personal hygiene.

What Your Kidneys Do For You:

- Help regulate blood pressure

- Adjust the amount of fluid in the body.

- Contribute to a proper pH balance vital to normal chemical reactions throughout the body. They re-absorb 90 percent of the filtered materials as a conservation measure.

- Remove blood toxins and non-storable excess nutrients or water.

- Help maintain proper sodium/potassium balance for more energy production.

Interesting Facts:

- The kidneys recycle about 45 gallons of blood every day.

- 25 percent of your blood is being filtered in the kidneys at any one time.

- Inside the kidneys are 2.4 million nephron filters requiring 50 miles of tiny capillaries and tubules.

Supplements for Urinary System Health
Irritated & Inflamed Urinary Tract:
Uva Ursi

Uva Ursi is used to treat cystitis—inflammation of the urinary tract. The main component of Uva Ursi is arbutin. Arbutin is absorbed in the stomach where it is converted into a substance with antimicrobial, astringent and antimicrobial properties.

Arbutin's main purpose is to soothe irritation and reduce inflammation during urination, as well as to fight infections in the urinary tract.

It is important for the urine to be alkaline for Uva Ursi to work properly. The acid / alkaline balance (pH) can be determined by using a litmus paper test strip. If the urine is too acidic then it can be brought to an alkaline state by the use of alkalizing agents such as calcium, magnesium supplements, chlorophyll in liquid form (chlorophyll is derived from alfalfa), and by eating alkalizing foods such as tomatoes, and the majority of fruits and vegetables. This is by no means a complete list. Note. While most citrus fruits are acidic, when they have been digested they are alkaline forming.

Acidic foods to avoid would include beef, pork, lamb, butter, peanut butter, to name a few. There are some excellent acid / alkaline food lists available on the Internet. Just type "acid alkaline food lists" into your search engine.

Marshmallow

This mucilant soothes the kidneys when they are irritated or inflamed. Marshmallow contains volatile oils and tannins that are responsible for its diuretic actions. It is especially helpful in passing kidney stones.

Urinary Tract Infections:
Cranberry

Cranberry's main purpose is to treat bacterial infections in the bladder. It is often combined with buchu herb.

When used together, these two herbs have anti-inflammatory, diuretic and antiseptic properties. Scientific studies show that cranberry makes the urinary tract inhospitable to bacteria, lessening the risk of urinary tract infections. Buchu acts as a diuretic and improves digestion. This product works best in acidic urine conditions.

Golden Seal

Golden seal has infection-fighting abilities and anti-inflammatory properties, and can be used as an alternative to cranberry if required.

Kidney Weakness:
Potassium

Potassium controls the balance of fluids in the body. In the urinary system it is used to treat water retention and various urinary problems. Consider taking a potassium supplement where there is a potassium deficiency due to excess flushing caused by urinary tract infections.

Horsetail

This herb has diuretic properties and can help with some kidney conditions. It is particularly effective for healing when blood is present in the urine. Horsetail also has astringent properties and as such, is used for bed-wetting in children and incontinence in Adults.

Horsetail is rich in silica, which helps to soothe and strengthen connective tissue. Silica is required for bone and cartilage formation, as well as assisting the body in absorbing and utilizing calcium. Calcium is required for repairing fractures and treating bone diseases, including rickets and osteoporosis. Horsetail is used to strengthen bones, teeth, nails and hair. Improvements in cartilage formation helps to lessen inflammation and combat joint pain, arthritis, gout, muscle cramps, hemorrhoids, spasms and rheumatism.

The silica content in horsetail also promotes the growth of collagen—a protein found in connective tissue, Collagen assists in improving skin health and tone.

Do You Live In a European Union Country

Of particular concern in Europe. In 2011 the European Union introduced the Herbal Medicines Directive which means the herbal industry has been all but destroyed by a draconian law which has all but banned the supply of herbal products within the European Union.

The excuse for issuing this directive is "to ensure public safety with regard to herbal products". I would have thought that something that has been used safely for hundreds (and in some cases thousands) of years would be safe for the public to take.

Many herbal products have been classified, not for use in food preparation (i.e. for cooking or garnishing purposes) but as "medicines" and a company now needs a license in order to sell them to the public. The cost of the license is in the order of $150,000 per herbal product. Yes, you read that correctly, $150,000 per herbal product.

Say you are a manufacturer and have just a small range of just 20 herbal products; that is going to cost you $3,000,000 in license fees, before you can sell anything. Very few manufacturers have that kind of money to waste on licenses for something that has been used safely for all those years.

All this new law is going to do is drive the supply of these safe, natural herbal products underground. With the power of modern communications and the Internet, all you have to do is spend a little time seeking out those herbal products you require from sources outside Europe. Many suppliers in other parts of the world—and especially the United States—will be more than happy to supply you, and will ship their products internationally. As the saying goes—where there's a will there's a way!!

Consult Your Doctor or a Naturopathic Doctor

In the body systems sections I have given you some product suggestions that have been used historically by herbalists and naturopaths for many years, but no suggested dosage requirements, or contra-indications.

The reason for this is that everyone is different. One person may need more of a particular product than the next person. Also, a particular product may suit one person, but not another.

Therefore I feel it is extremely important that you consult your doctor or a naturopathic doctor before commencing any supplement or herbal program, or changing your diet.

Additionally, you may be taking prescription medications for various health conditions which will, or could, have a negative impact on your health if you introduce vitamin or mineral supplements or a herbal program. Never take chances with your health.

I know that many doctors are not supportive of using a natural traditional route for health care. If your doctor feels this way and you would like to consider a more natural approach, then change your doctor and find one who is more supportive to your requirements.

About The Author

Brian B Jacques started in business when he was 11 years old, and over the ensuing years, he has developed several very successful businesses. But his main interest for the past 35 years has been in natural health research and book publishing.

He is a founding partner in Nature's Direct LLC a Florida, USA based supplier of nutritional supplements and herbal products, and Wisdom For Life Media, an online publisher of books which focus on the Health, Motivation and Personal Development fields. This company is also based in Florida, USA.

Brian has presented seminars worldwide on such diverse subjects as Health Related issues, Motivation and Personal Development. In addition he has written numerous books, newsletters and articles on these subjects.

His very popular series of Mini Health Books has circulated widely around the world, and many more titles are in preparation.

Brian is a highly motivated individual, so much so that in 1985 he received a UK Industrial Society award for his work in the Motivation and Personal Development fields.

Brian has the following mottos:

- If something does not work out for you, then don't give up, but keep trying, trying, trying until finally you succeed.
- Success or failure in any endeavor is in your own hands.

Brian was born in the UK and lives with his wife in Florida, USA, and East Yorkshire, UK.

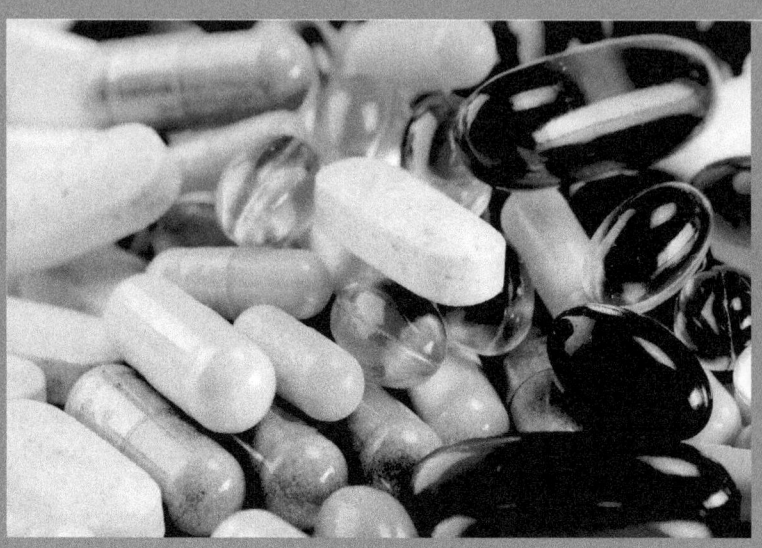

Index